Sildenafil (Viagra) for Men

The Comprehensive Guide Detailing Viagra Pills Usage for a Safe, Efficient, Long Lasting and Fast Acting Erection for Blue Sex and her Intimate Sensual Screaming Climax

Dr. Maya Mendoza

1

Copyright

[Dr. Maya Mendoza]

Table of Contents

Chapter One

Introduction

John had tried every treatment option he could think of for his erectile dysfunction, which had plagued him for years. No matter what drugs and vitamins he took, nothing appeared to work. Finally, his physician advised him to use Viagra.

John first had some reservations, but his doctor reassured him that it was secure and efficient. He reluctantly consented, but was taken aback by how rapidly it took effect. He saw a significant change in his capacity to achieve and sustain an erection within an hour of taking the medication.

His erectile issue ultimately disappeared totally as he continued to take Viagra. He was astounded by the medication's effectiveness and how well it had healed him. John may now enjoy a fulfilling and active sex life without worrying about his erectile problems.

Men with erectile dysfunction (ED) can be treated with Viagra, which is a prescription drug. It has been proven to be a safe and effective treatment for ED and is a drug that is frequently prescribed. Viagra helps men develop and maintain an erection by boosting blood flow to the penis. This drug comes in a variety of dosages and is administered orally. It is critical for medical experts and everyone to comprehend how Viagra functions, its negative effects, and the dosage that results in safe use. An overview of Viagra, its applications, key details, dosage, adverse reactions, storage, and a summary are provided in this manual.

Since its FDA approval in 1998, Viagra has grown to be one of the most widely used treatments for erectile dysfunction. Viagra comes in a variety of doses and is administered orally. The average Viagra dosage is 50 mg, although it can vary from 25 mg to 100 mg depending on the person.

Chapter Two

Dosage and Administration

Men with erectile dysfunction (ED) can be treated with Viagra. It functions by boosting blood flow to the penis, enabling men to get and keep an erection. The way Viagra works is by preventing the breakdown of a substance called cGMP by the enzyme PDE5. The blood flow to the penis is regulated by cGMP, and when it is suppressed, the blood vessels in the penis relax and broaden, enabling an increase in blood flow.

Viagra comes in a variety of doses and is administered orally. The starting dose of Viagra is 50 mg, which should be taken orally as needed about an hour before sexual activity. The dosage may be increased to 100 mg or decreased to 25 mg based on the person's response and tolerance. The highest daily dose that is advised is 100mg. Viagra shouldn't be taken more than once per day, and it shouldn't be combined with other drugs or alcoholic beverages.

Viagra should be taken orally with a glass of water about an hour prior to engaging in sexual activity. It can be taken with or without meals, although it is advised to stay away from a high-fat meal as this may cause the effects to take longer to manifest. You shouldn't take Viagra more than once a day.

To give Viagra enough time to work, it should be taken about an hour before engaging in sexual activity. After taking the drug, the effects of Viagra might persist for up to 4-5 hours.

When taken as prescribed, Viagra is a safe and efficient treatment for ED. Before using it, it's crucial to go over any possible dangers or side effects with your doctor. Headaches, flushing, stomach discomfort, and nasal congestion are typical Viagra adverse effects. More severe side effects may occasionally appear.

Chapter Three

Who should not take Viagra

Sildenafil, the active component in Viagra, should not be taken by anyone who has ever had an adverse reaction to sildenafil. People who are already on other medications, including nitrates or alpha-blockers, should also avoid using it because it can interact negatively with the effects of other drugs. People who have specific medical disorders, such as heart disease, kidney illness, or liver disease, should not take Viagra. These people should avoid using the medication.

Before beginning treatment with Viagra, it is essential to have a conversation with your primary care physician about any potential dangers or adverse effects. It is recommended that Viagra not be used more than once per day and that it not be combined with certain other drugs or alcohol. Men who have specific medical disorders, such as heart disease, renal illness, or liver disease, should also use

Viagra with caution before beginning treatment.

Chapter Four

Side Effects of Viagra

Men with erectile dysfunction (ED) can be treated with Viagra. It can enhance sexual function, but it can also have negative side effects. Headache, face flushing, dyspepsia, and nasal congestion are some of the most typical side effects of Viagra. These side effects are often mild to moderate in severity and disappear within a few hours or days. Some patients, however, can encounter more severe side effects that demand medical intervention.

The following are typical Viagra side effects:

Headaches: The most frequent side effect of Viagra is headache, which can happen in up to 16% of users. It can be mild to severe and may be brought on by the increased blood flow to the brain.

Facial Flushing: A typical Viagra adverse effect is facial flushing, which is characterized by redness, warmth, or tingling in the face or neck. Up to 10%

of people may have it, and it is often minor and temporary.

Indigestion: Symptoms of this adverse reaction include nausea, bloating, and discomfort in the abdomen. Up to 7% of people may have it, and it is often moderate and brief.

Nasal Congestion: Up to 4% of patients experience nasal congestion, which is characterized by a stuffy or runny nose. Usually, it is little and brief.

Dizziness: Up to 3% of individuals may experience the adverse effect of dizziness, which is characterized by a sense of faintness or lightheadedness. It might be brought on by the decline in blood pressure that might happen when using Viagra.

Vision Modifications: This adverse impact may include alterations in color perception, sensitivity to light, or blurred vision. It can affect up to 3% of patients and be brought on by variations in the blood flow to the eye.

Although they are uncommon, serious Viagra side effects can include:

Sudden Hearing Loss: A rare but dangerous side effect that can happen to some patients is sudden hearing loss. It might be brought on by a reduction in blood supply to the ear, and if it is not treated right once, it can cause permanent hearing loss.

Sudden Vision Loss: Another uncommon but significant side effect of using Viagra is sudden vision loss. It might be brought on by a reduction in blood flow to the optic nerve, and if it is not treated right once, it can cause permanent vision loss.

Priapism: When an erection lasts more than four hours, an uncommon but significant side effect known as priapism might occur. It might hurt and need medical attention to get well.

Severe Allergic Reactions: These can include hives, trouble breathing, swelling of the face, lips, tongue, or neck. Although uncommon, these reactions have the potential to be fatal.

Cardiovascular Events: In some people with a history of cardiovascular illness, using Viagra has been linked to an elevated risk of cardiovascular events, such as a heart attack or stroke.

Before using Viagra, patients should talk to their doctor about their medical history, any potential risks, and any possible adverse effects. If they encounter any severe or lingering side effects while using Viagra, they should also contact a doctor.

Chapter Five

Managing Side Effects

Men with erectile dysfunction can take the drug to address their condition. Although not everyone will have negative effects, Viagra can cause them just like any other medication. Headache, face flushing, nasal congestion, dyspepsia, and visual abnormalities are some of the most frequent side effects of Viagra.

Here are some suggestions for managing the adverse effects of Viagra:

Headache: A typical Viagra side effect is a headache. Patients can take over-the-counter pain relievers like acetaminophen or ibuprofen to treat headaches. Patients should consult their healthcare provider if headaches continue.

Facial Flushing: A typical adverse effect of Viagra is facial flushing, which happens when blood vessels in the face enlarge. Patients can manage facial flushing by avoiding triggers like alcohol and spicy foods. Water consumption might also aid in symptom relief.

Nasal Congestion: Another typical side effect of Viagra is nasal congestion. Nasal decongestants sold without a prescription can be used by patients to ease symptoms. To avoid rebound congestion, patients should refrain from using nasal decongestants for longer than three days.

Indigestion: One of Viagra's common side effects is indigestion. By eating smaller, more often meals and staying away from fatty or spicy foods, patients can manage indigestion. Additionally, patients have access to over-the-counter antacids for symptom relief.

Vision changes: Blurred vision and altered color perception are uncommon Viagra adverse effects. Patients who encounter any vision abnormalities while taking Viagra should visit a doctor right once.

It is crucial for people to discuss any negative effects they have while using Viagra with their doctor. To manage side effects, it may occasionally be required to adjust the dosage or medication. Additionally, patients should adhere to the dosage guidelines given by their doctor and refrain from ingesting more Viagra than is advised.

Chapter Six

Interactions

Viagra (sildenafil citrate) might interact with other medicines or foods, perhaps resulting in negative side effects or lowering the medication's effectiveness. Before taking Viagra, patients should talk with their doctor about their current pharmaceutical regimen and eating habits to rule out any potential interactions.

Drugs that frequently interact with Viagra include:

a. **Nitrates:** Nitrates are drugs that cure heart failure or chest pain. They can reduce blood pressure because they function by widening the blood arteries. Nitrates and Viagra together can cause a significant reduction in blood pressure that is potentially fatal. If a patient is using nitrates like nitroglycerin, isosorbide dinitrate, or isosorbide mononitrate, they shouldn't take Viagra.

b. **Alpha-blockers:** These drugs are used to treat excessive blood pressure or symptoms of an enlarged prostate that affect the urinary system. They can reduce blood pressure because they function by loosening the blood vessel muscles. Alpha-blockers and Viagra together can cause a significant reduction in blood pressure that is potentially fatal. Before taking Viagra, patients who use alpha-blockers should talk to their doctor about their prescription regimen.

c. **Protease Inhibitors:** Drugs called protease inhibitors are used to treat AIDS and HIV. They may raise the blood levels of Viagra, which could increase the chance of adverse effects. Before taking Viagra, patients who use protease inhibitors should talk to their doctor about their prescription usage.

d. **Other erectile dysfunction drugs:**

Patients should not use more than one erectile dysfunction drug at once, including Viagra and Cialis (tadalafil). Combining these drugs may not provide any additional advantages and may increase the risk of negative effects.

Viagra can interact with specific foods in addition to medications, including:

a. **Grapefruit and Grapefruit Juice:** Grapefruit can raise the blood levels of Viagra, which could increase the chance of adverse effects. While taking Viagra, patients should refrain from drinking grapefruit or grapefruit juice.

b. **High-fat meals:** Eating a high-fat meal just before taking Viagra can make it less effective. For best effectiveness, patients should take Viagra on an empty stomach or right after a small meal.

Before taking Viagra, patients should let their doctor know whether they take any drugs, dietary supplements, or other supplements. While using

Viagra, they should also refrain from consuming alcohol and using recreational drugs because these activities can interact with the pill and have unfavorable effects.

Chapter Seven
Precautions

Patients should talk to their doctor about their medical history and any current drugs they are taking before taking Viagra (sildenafil citrate). Here are some safety measures to follow when taking Viagra:

- **Medical history:** Before taking Viagra, patients with a history of heart disease, stroke, or low blood pressure should talk to their doctor about their health history. Patients with low blood pressure should use Viagra cautiously because it can drop blood pressure.
- **Allergies:** Individuals with allergies to sildenafil or any other component of Viagra should avoid taking the drug.
- **Medication:** Patients should disclose all drugs

they are currently taking to their healthcare provider, including prescription, over-the-counter, dietary supplements, and herbal therapies. Alpha-blockers, protease inhibitors, nitrates, and other medicines can interact with Viagra and have negative side effects.

- **Alcohol and Recreational Drugs:** Patients taking Viagra should abstain from drinking alcohol and using recreational drugs. These chemicals may interact with the drug and raise the possibility of negative side effects.

- **Grapefruit and Grapefruit Juice:** Patients on Viagra should refrain from drinking grapefruit or grapefruit juice. The blood levels of Viagra can rise when grapefruit is consumed, thus increasing the risk of adverse effects.

- **Driving and Operating Machinery:** Patients on Viagra may have dizziness and vision problems, which may impair their ability to do either. Patients should refrain from using machinery or driving until they are familiar with how Viagra affects them.

- **Priapism:** The usage of Viagra may result in an erection that lasts longer than four hours. Patients who develop an erection that lasts longer than four hours should contact a doctor right away.

Viagra is not advised for usage by women during pregnancy or while nursing. The medication's effects on the fetus or a breastfed child are unknown because it has not been researched in pregnant or nursing women.

It is crucial for people to adhere to their doctor's dosage recommendations and refrain from taking more Viagra than is advised. Additionally, patients should visit a doctor if they suffer any adverse effects or have any worries while taking the medicine.

Chapter Eight

Viagra Overdose

Sildenafil citrate, the active ingredient in Viagra, can be taken in excess and cause harmful adverse effects. It's crucial to take Viagra exactly as directed by a doctor and to refrain from exceeding the advised dosage. In the event of an overdose, prompt medical care is required. In order to treat a Viagra overdose, follow these steps:

i. **Contact emergency services:** If a person has taken more Viagra than is advised, contact emergency services or get to the closest medical room right away. In the event of an overdose, time is of the importance.

ii. **Symptoms:** Severe dizziness, fainting, chest pain, an irregular heartbeat, and changes in eyesight can all be signs of a Viagra overdose. Priapism, an erection that lasts longer than four hours, can also occur in patients. Priapism may be a medical emergency that needs to be treated right away.

iii. **Treatment:** If you take too much Viagra, you may need to have your stomach pumped to get rid of any leftover drug. You may also need to take medicine to treat symptoms like low blood pressure or an irregular pulse, as well as receive supportive care like oxygen treatment. Treatment for priapism may involve draining blood from the penis or giving patients drugs that relax blood vessels and lower blood flow.

iv. **Prevention:** To prevent a Viagra overdose, patients should adhere to the dosage recommendations given by their doctor and abstain from exceeding them. Additionally, patients should abstain from consuming alcohol or recreational drugs while using Viagra because these substances raise the possibility of overdose and adverse effects.

If you take too much Viagra, you should seek medical help right away. To avoid interactions and possible overdose, patients should also let their doctor know about any medications they are taking, including over-the-counter drugs, vitamins, and herbal remedies. In order to lower the risk of adverse effects and overdose, patients should also heed the warnings and precautions given by their healthcare professional before taking Viagra.

Chapter Nine
Storage of Viagra

To preserve its efficacy and safety, Viagra (sildenafil citrate) should be stored appropriately. The following are instructions on how to properly store Viagra:

a. **Temperature:** Viagra should be kept between

68°F and 77°F (20°C and 25°C) at room temperature. Direct sunshine, heat, and wetness should all be avoided. Keep Viagra away from humid areas like the kitchen or bathroom where it can be exposed.

b. **Packaging:** Until it is time to use it, Viagra should be kept in its original container. The packaging aids in shielding the medication from light and moisture, two factors that could cause the medication to deteriorate and lose some of its potency.

c. Pets and children should not have access to Viagra, which should be kept out of their reach. Accidental ingestion of the drug should be prevented because it might be harmful if consumed by kids or animals.

d. Viagra should be appropriately disposed of if it is no longer required or has expired. Viagra should not be dumped down the drain or flushed down the toilet. Ask your neighborhood pharmacy or waste management center for the right disposal procedures.

e. Viagra should be kept in a safe, cool location while traveling, such as a carry-on luggage. Viagra shouldn't be kept in checked luggage because it can be subjected to extreme humidity and temperature changes when traveling.

For Viagra to be safe and effective, it must be stored properly. Before taking a drug, patients should always check the expiration date to make sure it is still valid. Patients should ask their doctor or pharmacist for advice if they have any worries or queries regarding how to store Viagra.

Chapter Ten

Conclusion

In conclusion, Viagra (sildenafil citrate) is a successful drug that is frequently recommended to treat erectile dysfunction. When applied correctly, it can enhance patients' quality of life and sexual performance. However, it is crucial to use Viagra responsibly and adhere to the dosing guidelines given by a healthcare professional. Additionally, patients need to be informed about possible adverse effects, medication interactions, and safety measures to follow when taking Viagra. Patients should also appropriately store their medications and dispose of them when they are no longer needed. Patients should get advice from their doctor or pharmacist if they have any worries or inquiries about using Viagra. Patients who adhere to these recommendations and use

Viagra sensibly can treat erectile dysfunction safely and effectively.

The End

Made in the USA
Monee, IL
28 May 2023

34798170R10028